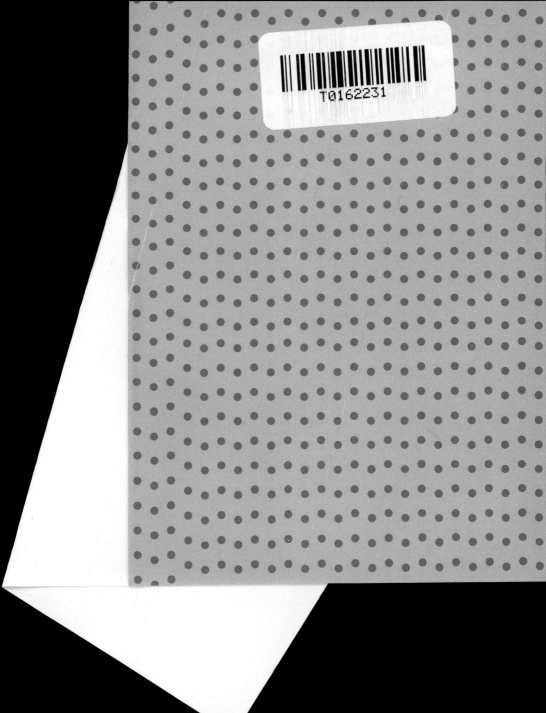

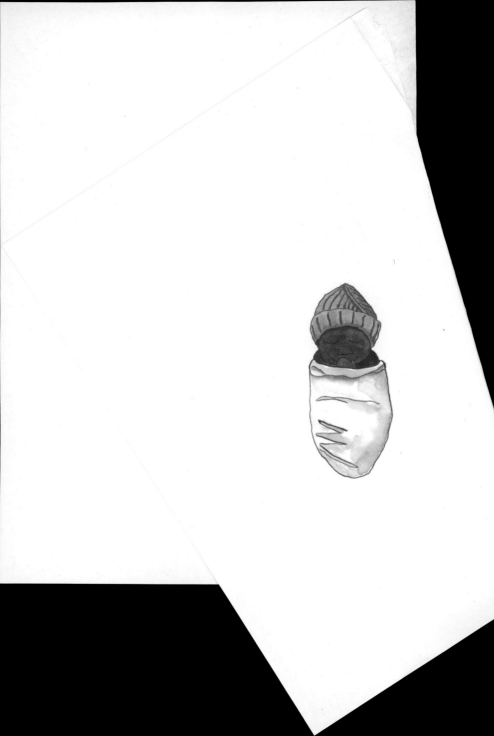

# A Bun in the Oven

### A weekly guide to the wonders of pregnancy

Written and illustrated by
## Hannah Hunter-Kelm

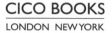

**CICO BOOKS**
LONDON NEW YORK

This edition published in 2020 by CICO Books
An imprint of Ryland Peters & Small Ltd
20–21 Jockey's Fields, London WC1R 4BW
341 E 116th St, New York NY 10029

www.rylandpeters.com

10 9 8 7 6 5 4 3 2 1

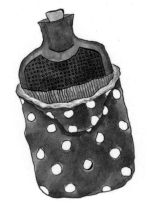

Editor: Jane Perlmutter
Design concept: Hannah Hunter-Kelm
Designer: Jerry Goldie

Senior editor: Carmel Edmonds
Art director: Sally Powell
Head of production: Patricia Harrington
Publishing manager: Penny Craig
Publisher: Cindy Richards

A CIP catalog record for this book is available
from the Library of Congress and the
British Library.

ISBN: 978-1-78249-825-4

Printed in China

## PLEASE NOTE

All size comparisons are approximate—after
all, every baby is different. The advice in
this book is not considered to be a substitute
for medical advice from your family
physician or doctor or any other qualified
medical practitioner.

# Contents

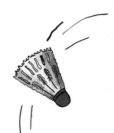

# Introduction

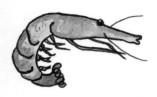 The idea for this week-by-week guide came about when I was working in a healthcare office with a lovely bunch of ladies. When one of my co-workers announced that she was pregnant, there was endless speculation about potential names and how fast the baby was growing in the womb. Turning to the Internet for guidance on fetus sizes, I was perplexed by websites which compared this new life to a series of vegetables that I had never heard of, let alone could visualize. In that moment,

the idea of an alternative pregnancy calendar was conceived. The drawings throughout this book have been made using my left hand (not my natural hand) to give them a childlike quality. My hope is that this little book will fill you with wonder (and useful information) as you progress through your pregnancy.

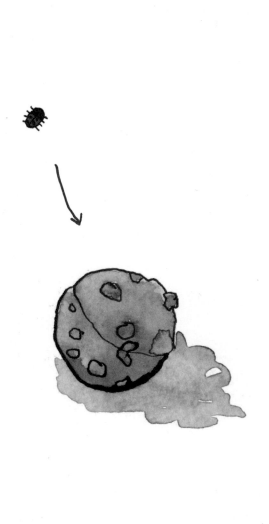

# FIRST TRIMESTER

## Weeks 6–12

### From Ladybug
### to Bath Bomb

## TOP TIP:
To help your baby grow and
develop, eat foods that are rich
in calcium, vitamin C, iron, and
folic acid (like cereal,
eggs, red meat, yummy green
veggies, and chickpeas).

# Week 6

Your baby is the size of a
## ladybug.

(In other words, teeny tiny!)

# Week 7

INTERESTING FACT:
Hands and feet that look like
tiny paddles have appeared.

You have a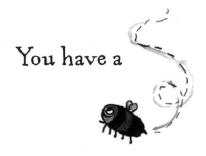

bumblebee-sized baby!

# Week 8

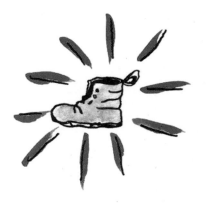

This week your baby
is the size of the
Monopoly boot.

You may experience
morning sickness.

## SORRY!

Ginger tea, ginger snaps,
or crystallized ginger might help.

# Week 9

**INTERESTING FACT:**
Tiny eyelids cover your baby's eyes,
but they won't open until week 26!

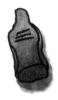

Your baby is now as big as one of those **cola-bottle candies.**

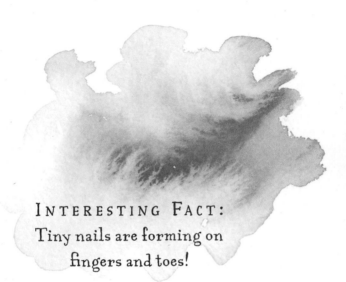

**INTERESTING FACT:**
Tiny nails are forming on
fingers and toes!

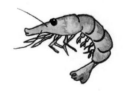

# Week 10

Your baby is just over
1¼in./3.1cm long.

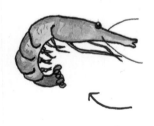

(About as big as
a medium-sized
shrimpy shrimp.)

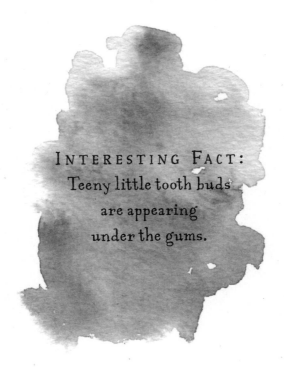

INTERESTING FACT:
Teeny little tooth buds
are appearing
under the gums.

# Week 11

Your baby is the length of
a tube of lipstick...

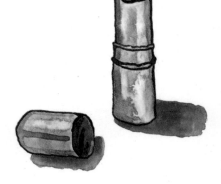

just over
1½in./4cm
long.

# Week 12

TOP TIP:
This week is a good week to start
doing some pelvic floor (Kegel)
exercises. (How about every time
you wait for the kettle
to boil for tea?)

Around this week, you'll have
an ultrasound scan which will
give you your official
Estimated Due Date (EDD).

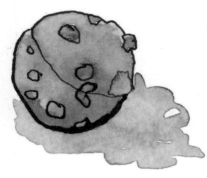

Your baby is
now the size

of a mini
bath bomb.

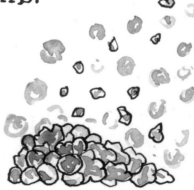

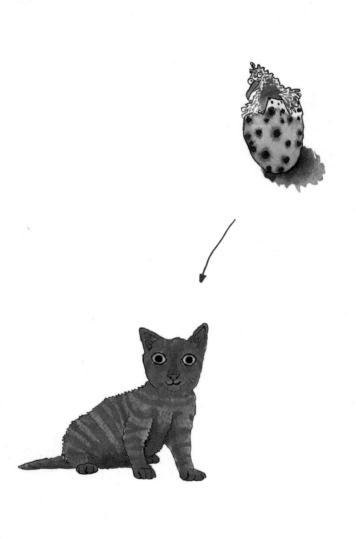

# SECOND TRIMESTER

## Weeks 13–27

From Seagull Egg
to Kitten

# Week 13

At the moment, your baby only weighs about ¾oz/21g!

↑

(The same as a pea pod.)

Your baby is the size
of a **seagull egg**
(about 2¾in./7cm).

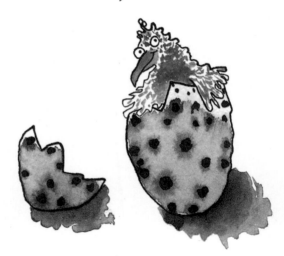

# Week 14

INTERESTING FACT:
Your baby can now suck
his/her thumb!

Computer mouse

Currently about
the same length as
your future
son/daughter!

# Week 15

At roughly 3½in./9.1cm
long, your baby is about
the same size as a

badminton shuttlecock (birdie).

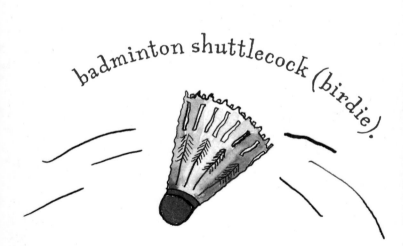

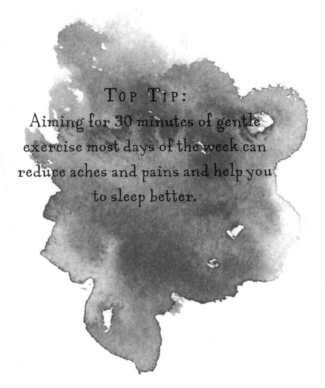

TOP TIP:
Aiming for 30 minutes of gentle
exercise most days of the week can
reduce aches and pains and help you
to sleep better.

INTERESTING FACT:
Over the next few weeks
your baby's weight will

double!

# Week 16

Imagine a
**glue stick**
–that's the length
of your baby!

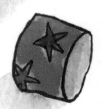

TOP TIP:
Your eyes might start
feeling a bit dry. If so,
eye drops might help.

# Week 17

If you make yourself some toast
with jelly this week, imagine
your baby is the
size of the
jelly jar!

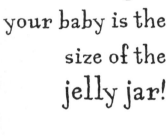

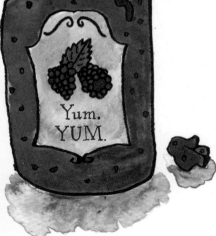

Yum.
YUM.

# Week 18

Remember these?

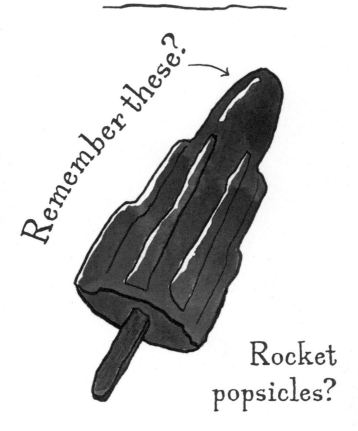

Rocket popsicles?

One popsicle is about
the length of your
baby this week.

You may feel your baby
kicking and wriggling
around, although some
women don't feel first
movements until week 22.

# Week 19

Some research says your baby may be able to hear you now—how about reading him/her a story?

This week your baby is about the size of a mini coffee press!

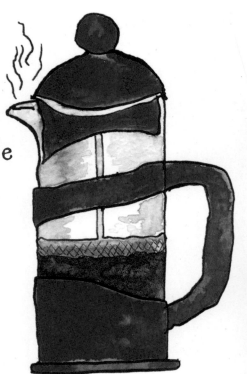

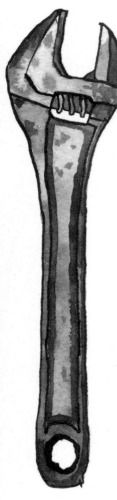

# Week 20

Your baby is growing like a champ! At 10¼in./26cm long, he/she is the length of a wrench or spanner.

(From this point on, babies are usually measured from crown to heel rather than crown to rump.)

Around this week you'll have your
ultrasound scan (to check that your baby is
developing normally). It is also a chance to
find out if you're having a boy or a girl!

INTERESTING FACT:
You will probably gain about
1lb/500g a week from now on.
(Not forever, just until the birth!)

# Week 21

The purchase of ~~½~~ 2
## chocolate éclairs
is <u>essential</u> to visualizing the
length of
your baby this week.

No excuses, please.

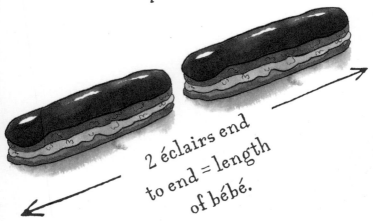

2 éclairs end to end = length of bébé.

# Week 22

At roughly 11in./28cm, your baby is starting to look like a miniature newborn.

Curled up, he/she would be about the size of a butter dish.

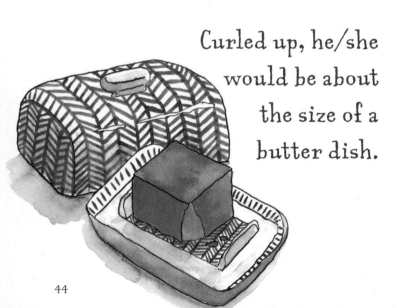

You may start
to experience
s t r e t c h
marks.


TOP TIP:
Moisturizer might
help with any itching.

# Week 23

Have your ankles turned
into cankles?
Don't worry—swollen
ankles are normal at
this stage.

Weighing just over 1lb/500g, your baby is now about the size of a guinea pig, but has less fur.

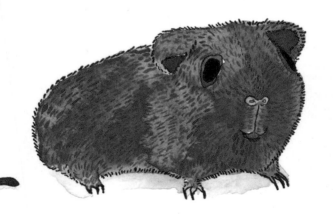

# Week 24

Your baby has put on about
4oz/110g in one week, and
now somewhat resembles the
size of a cheese grater.

INTERESTING FACT:
Your baby's inner ear organs
are currently developing.

HAVE A GRATE WEEK!

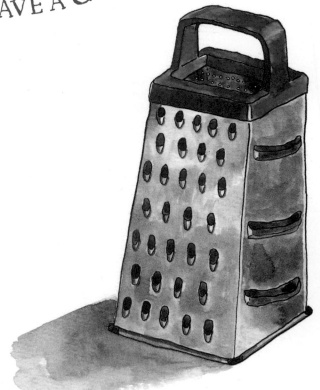

# Week 25

INTERESTING FACT:
Your baby's hair is growing, and
yours might look fuller and

shinier

at this point.

Your baby is about 13¾ in./
35cm from top to bottom,
but if he/she curled into
a ball it would be
about the size of a...

GREAT BIG hairy coconut.

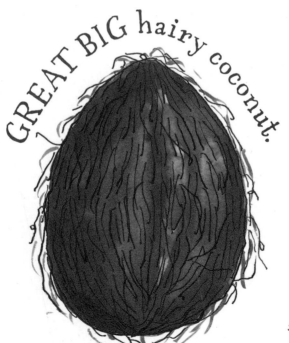

TOP TIP:
Ask your doctor or midwife
about prenatal (antenatal)
classes (also called childbirth
or Parentcraft Classes)—most
start 8–10 weeks before your
due date. They can be a great
way to learn more about the
birthing process and how to
take care of your baby.

# Week 26

Ever play the recorder
when you were younger?
At 14⅛in./36cm, it's
about the length of
your baby when he/she
**s t r e t c h e s** out.

Your baby's eyelids
will start to open
this week!

# Week 27

This week, your baby is about the size of an 8-week-old kitten, and weighs around 2lb/900g.

Has your belly button popped out yet?!

CUUUTE!

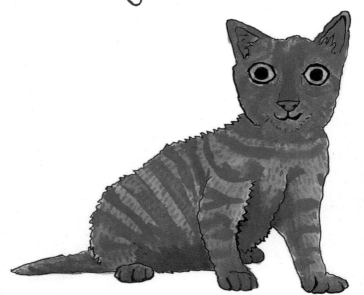

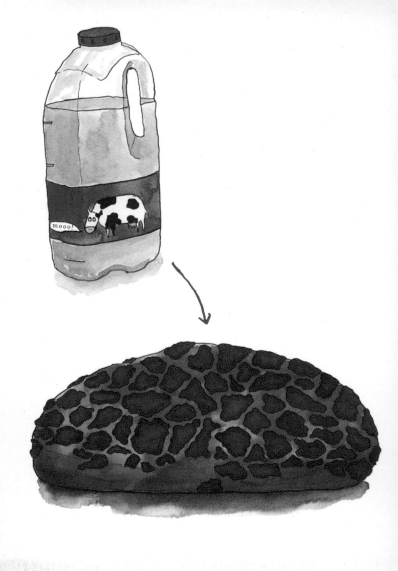

# THIRD TRIMESTER

# Weeks 28–40
From Milk Carton
to Large Loaf

# Week 28

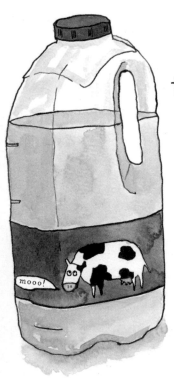

You've reached your **third trimester!** At around 15in./ 38cm, your baby is similar to the size of a half-gallon/4-pint **carton** of **milk.**

By now, you will have noticed your baby kicking more. Keep a record of your baby's normal movement pattern—if you notice any change in it, call your doctor or midwife.

TOP TIP:
Try a HOT or COOL pack if your lower back is feeling achey.

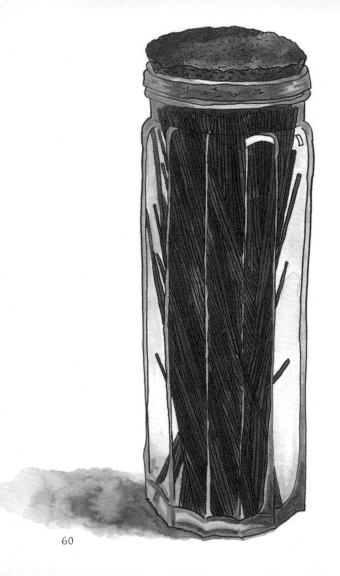

# Week 29

Feeling **extra** hungry
this week?
Why not make some pasta?
Your happy "wee bundle"
is about the same size
as a spaghetti jar.

The large majority of babies react
to light and sounds by the end
of this week. You may even feel
your baby **jump** at loud noises!

# Week 30

Does your baby feel like a **sports superstar** in the making?

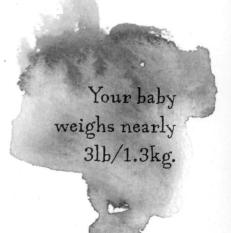

Your baby weighs nearly 3lb/1.3kg.

This week, he/she is roughly the same size as a

football!

↓

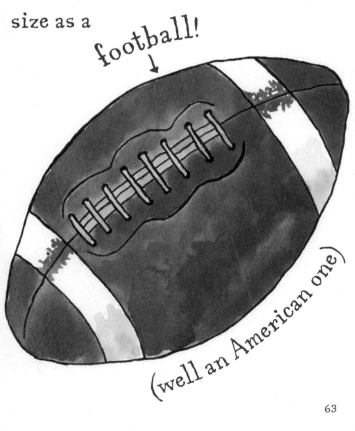

(well an American one)

# Get Ready to Shop!

Use these checklists to ensure you have everything you'll need for your newborn.

## TRAVEL

- [ ] Car seat/travel system
- [ ] Stroller that lies flat, if not part of the travel system
- [ ] Stroller accessories, such as a rain cover and/or sun shade
- [ ] Baby carrier (optional)

## SLEEPING

- [ ] Bassinet/Moses basket/carrycot and mattress
- [ ] Crib/cot and mattress
- [ ] Sheets and blankets
- [ ] Baby sleeping bag (optional)

- [ ] Baby monitor
- [ ] Mobile (optional)

## NAPPIES

- [ ] Disposable diapers/nappies
- [ ] Diaper/nappy sacks
- [ ] Lotions and wipes
- [ ] Changing table and mat
- [ ] Changing bag
- [ ] Cloth diapers/Muslins

For reusable diapers/nappies, you will need liners, sterilizer, and a bucket. You may want to keep some disposables for emergencies.

## BATHING

- [ ] Baby bath or bath support that can be used in the main bath
- [ ] Baby towels (optional)
- [ ] Mild baby cleanser
- [ ] Cotton wool

## IF YOU'RE PLANNING TO BREASTFEED

- [ ] Nursing bras
- [ ] Breast pads
- [ ] Nipple cream
- [ ] Breast pump (optional)

## IF YOU'RE PLANNING TO BOTTLE-FEED

- [ ] Sterilizer or another sterilizing method
- [ ] Bottles and brushes

Even if you're planning to breastfeed, it's handy to have this equipment from birth so that you have the option of bottle-feeding expressed breast milk.

## NEWBORN CLOTHES

- [ ] Onesies/Babygros (at least 8)
- [ ] Bodysuits/Vests (at least 8)
- [ ] Bibs
- [ ] Cardigans
- [ ] Socks
- [ ] Hat, depending on the season
- [ ] Coat/all-in-one suit, depending on the season
- [ ] Thermometer

## OTHER USEFUL EQUIPMENT

- [ ] Bouncy chair
- [ ] Baby playmat
- [ ] High chair (from 6 months)

# Week 31

Your baby is around
16in./41cm
from top to toe.

If you are lucky enough to come across an ENORMOUS

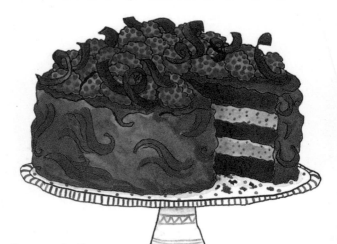

chocolate cake
this week, then
it might well be the size
and weight of your baby!

# Week 32

This week your
"wee babby" is roughly
the size of a lovely,
snuggly hot water
bottle.

INTERESTING FACT:
Your baby is now peeing
about a pint/0.5 liters
every day!
YUM!

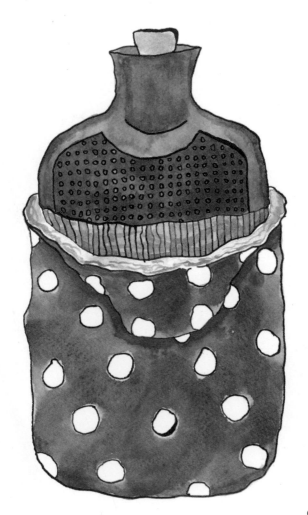

# Week 33

Imagine a bonsai tree
17¼in./44cm high.

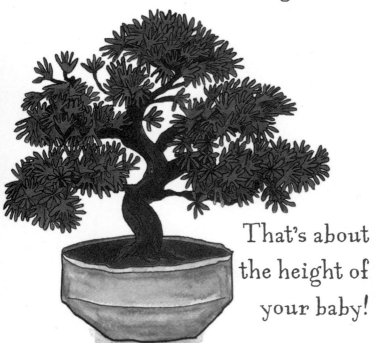

That's about
the height of
your baby!

Ready to prepare for his/her entrance into **the world**, your baby may have already turned upside down.

# Week 34

TOP TIP:
This week is a good
time to start making
your birth plan.

Time for a new handbag?
When you hit the stores,
you'll be looking at the
approximate size
of your baby
this week.

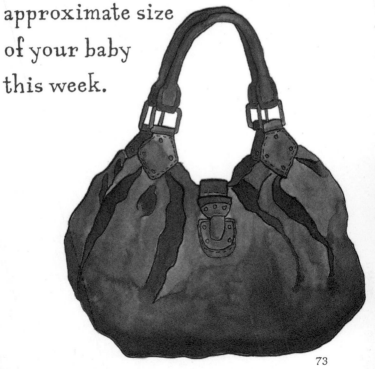

# Week 35

TOP TIP:
You are likely to feel
tired—remember to
take it easy!

Having a BUOY?
(You get my drift...)

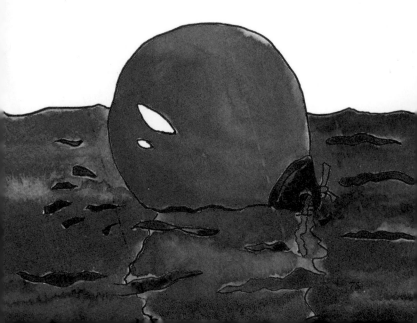

# Hospital Bag Checklist

Even if you're planning a home birth, it's worth packing a bag a few weeks in advance of the due date in case of an emergency.

☐ Birth plan
☐ Maternity notes

## CLOTHING

☐ Old T-Shirt or nightgown
☐ Dressing gown
☐ Thongs/flip-flops or slippers
☐ Underwear
☐ Clothes to go home
☐ Front-opening tops to breastfeed

## TOILETRIES

☐ Usual toiletries, plus massage oil and lip balm to use in labor, if you wish, and hair clips/ties for long hair

## SNACKS AND DRINKS

☐ Your birth partner can buy them for you at the hospital, but it's worth taking along things you find particularly refreshing and energizing

## ITEMS TO PASS THE TIME

☐ Music, magazines, books, tablet

## LABOR ACCESSORIES

☐ A birth ball, if planning to use

☐ TENS machine, if planning to use

## FOR AFTER THE BIRTH

☐ Nursing bras

☐ Breast pads

☐ Maternity pads

## FOR YOUR NEWBORN

☐ Nappies

☐ Cloth diapers/ muslins

☐ Onesies/babygros and bodysuits/vests

☐ Socks

☐ A going-home outfit, plus coat, hat, and blanket depending on the season

☐ Baby car seat

# Week 36

This week your baby
is about the length

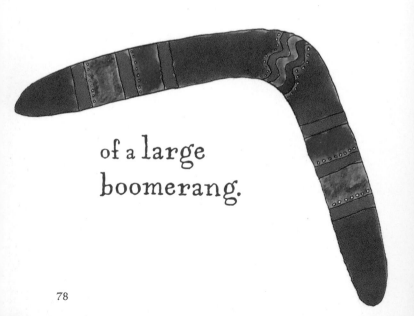

of a large
boomerang.

If you're having twins,
you're nearly done!
Around half of twins
are born at the end of
36 weeks.

At around
19in./48cm,
your baby
is about
the height
of a pair of
boots.

# Week 37

Do you have a list
of favorite
names yet?

# The Name Game

Choosing a name for your baby can be daunting, but fun! Use these lists to jot down the names you like and, hopefully, you can get down to at least a short-list of three before the big day!

BOYS' NAMES:
LONG-LIST                    MEANING

1......................................    ..................................................

2......................................    ..................................................

3......................................    ..................................................

4......................................    ..................................................

5......................................    ..................................................

6......................................    ..................................................

7......................................    ..................................................

8......................................    ..................................................

9......................................    ..................................................

10....................................    ..................................................

## GIRLS' NAMES:
## LONG-LIST

### MEANING

1.................................... ....................................

2.................................... ....................................

3.................................... ....................................

4.................................... ....................................

5.................................... ....................................

6.................................... ....................................

7.................................... ....................................

8.................................... ....................................

9.................................... ....................................

10.................................. ....................................

## GIRLS' NAMES:
SHORT-LIST

## BOYS' NAMES:
SHORT-LIST

1.................................... 1....................................

2.................................... 2....................................

3.................................... 3....................................

# Week 38

You're so nearly there!
Your baby is about the length
of a snorkel, and almost
ready to say

# hello!

He/she is busy putting
on a layer of fat to keep warm
and toasty outside the womb.

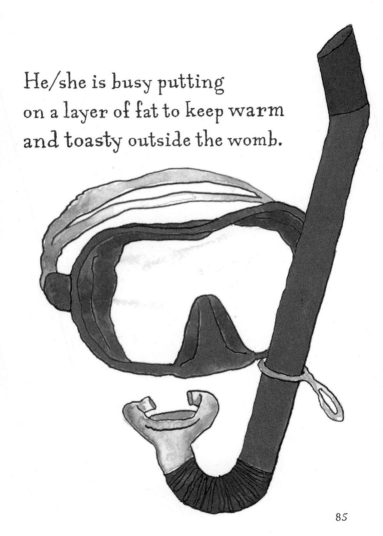

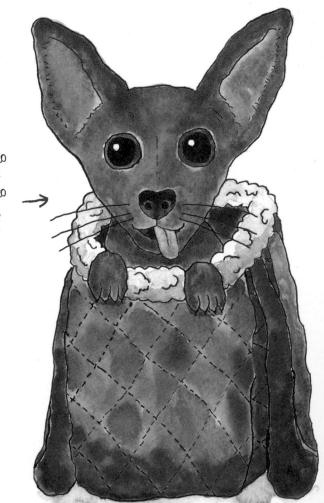

a. k. a. handbag dog

# Week 39

Measuring about
19½in./50cm, this week
your baby is about the size
of a chihuahua, but much
better looking!

# Week 40

This week you truly do have a bun in the oven: your baby is approximately the size of...

a large loaf of crusty bread.

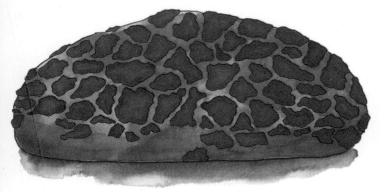

# GO FORTH AND GIVE BIRTH, AMAZING WOMAN!

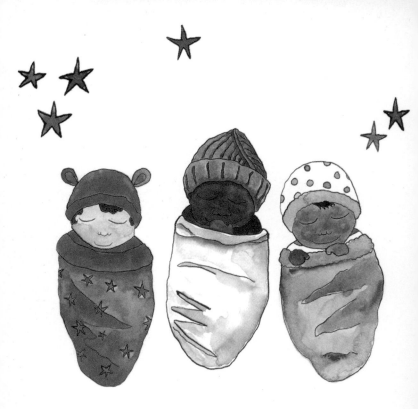

WELL DONE!

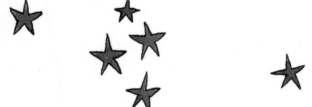

# Pregnancy
# Calendar

## JANUARY

| 1 | 2 | 3 | 4 | 5 | 6 | 7 |
|---|---|---|---|---|---|---|
| 8 | 9 | 10 | 11 | 12 | 13 | 14 |
| 15 | 16 | 17 | 18 | 19 | 20 | 21 |
| 22 | 23 | 24 | 25 | 26 | 27 | 28 |
| 29 | 30 | 31 | | | | |

## FEBRUARY

| 1 | 2 | 3 | 4 | 5 | 6 | 7 |
|---|---|---|---|---|---|---|
| 8 | 9 | 10 | 11 | 12 | 13 | 14 |
| 15 | 16 | 17 | 18 | 19 | 20 | 21 |
| 22 | 23 | 24 | 25 | 26 | 27 | 28 |
| 29 | | | | | | |

## MARCH

| 1 | 2 | 3 | 4 | 5 | 6 | 7 |
|---|---|---|---|---|---|---|
| 8 | 9 | 10 | 11 | 12 | 13 | 14 |
| 15 | 16 | 17 | 18 | 19 | 20 | 21 |
| 22 | 23 | 24 | 25 | 26 | 27 | 28 |
| 29 | 30 | 31 | | | | |

Use this calendar to keep a note of your
hospital appointments, prenatal classes and,
of course, your due date!

APRIL

| 1 | 2 | 3 | 4 | 5 | 6 | 7 |
|---|---|---|---|---|---|---|
| 8 | 9 | 10 | 11 | 12 | 13 | 14 |
| 15 | 16 | 17 | 18 | 19 | 20 | 21 |
| 22 | 23 | 24 | 25 | 26 | 27 | 28 |
| 29 | 30 | | | | | |

MAY

| 1 | 2 | 3 | 4 | 5 | 6 | 7 |
|---|---|---|---|---|---|---|
| 8 | 9 | 10 | 11 | 12 | 13 | 14 |
| 15 | 16 | 17 | 18 | 19 | 20 | 21 |
| 22 | 23 | 24 | 25 | 26 | 27 | 28 |
| 29 | 30 | 31 | | | | |

JUNE

| 1 | 2 | 3 | 4 | 5 | 6 | 7 |
|---|---|---|---|---|---|---|
| 8 | 9 | 10 | 11 | 12 | 13 | 14 |
| 15 | 16 | 17 | 18 | 19 | 20 | 21 |
| 22 | 23 | 24 | 25 | 26 | 27 | 28 |
| 29 | 30 | | | | | |

## JULY

| 1 | 2 | 3 | 4 | 5 | 6 | 7 |
|---|---|---|---|---|---|---|
| 8 | 9 | 10 | 11 | 12 | 13 | 14 |
| 15 | 16 | 17 | 18 | 19 | 20 | 21 |
| 22 | 23 | 24 | 25 | 26 | 27 | 28 |
| 29 | 30 | 31 | | | | |

## AUGUST

| 1 | 2 | 3 | 4 | 5 | 6 | 7 |
|---|---|---|---|---|---|---|
| 8 | 9 | 10 | 11 | 12 | 13 | 14 |
| 15 | 16 | 17 | 18 | 19 | 20 | 21 |
| 22 | 23 | 24 | 25 | 26 | 27 | 28 |
| 29 | 30 | 31 | | | | |

## SEPTEMBER

| 1 | 2 | 3 | 4 | 5 | 6 | 7 |
|---|---|---|---|---|---|---|
| 8 | 9 | 10 | 11 | 12 | 13 | 14 |
| 15 | 16 | 17 | 18 | 19 | 20 | 21 |
| 22 | 23 | 24 | 25 | 26 | 27 | 28 |
| 29 | 30 | | | | | |

## OCTOBER

| 1 | 2 | 3 | 4 | 5 | 6 | 7 |
|---|---|---|---|---|---|---|
| 8 | 9 | 10 | 11 | 12 | 13 | 14 |
| 15 | 16 | 17 | 18 | 19 | 20 | 21 |
| 22 | 23 | 24 | 25 | 26 | 27 | 28 |
| 29 | 30 | 31 | | | | |

## NOVEMBER

| 1 | 2 | 3 | 4 | 5 | 6 | 7 |
|---|---|---|---|---|---|---|
| 8 | 9 | 10 | 11 | 12 | 13 | 14 |
| 15 | 16 | 17 | 18 | 19 | 20 | 21 |
| 22 | 23 | 24 | 25 | 26 | 27 | 28 |
| 29 | 30 | | | | | |

## DECEMBER

| 1 | 2 | 3 | 4 | 5 | 6 | 7 |
|---|---|---|---|---|---|---|
| 8 | 9 | 10 | 11 | 12 | 13 | 14 |
| 15 | 16 | 17 | 18 | 19 | 20 | 21 |
| 22 | 23 | 24 | 25 | 26 | 27 | 28 |
| 29 | 30 | 31 | | | | |

# Acknowledgments

This book is dedicated to the wonderful admin ladies who I worked with at the NHS office, Shaftesbury House, Leeds, in 2011/2012 and particularly to Paula Simpson, whose pregnancy inspired this idea. Also, to my nephews who inspired me to get drawing—Joshua, Finn, Ezra, Rory, and Gus—but especially to our own "buns in the oven," Jago and Saskia. Big thanks to my amazing husband, Jonny, my brilliant family, and all the friends who have inspired me and helped out practically with this project.

Finally, I'm in awe of the One who thought up the miracle of conception, pregnancy, and birth—The Creator and Giver of Life.

Because:

"You created every part of me;

You put me together in my mother's womb."

Psalm 139, Verse 13

(The *Good News* translation of the Bible)